Fight Fatigue

A Training Handbook for Nurses

HCPro

Fight Fatigue: A Training Handbook for Nurses is published by HCPro, Inc.

ISBN 1-57839-544-5

HCPro, Inc. provides information resources for the healthcare industry.

Adrianne E. Avillion, DEd, RN, Author
John Gettings, Managing Editor
Jean St. Pierre, Creative Director
Mike Mirabello, Senior Graphic Artist
Laura Godinho, Cover Designer
Emily Sheahan, Executive Editor
Kathy Levesque, Group Publisher
Suzanne Perney, Publisher

For more information, contact:

HCPro, Inc.
200 Hoods Lane
P.O. Box 1168
Marblehead, MA 01945
Telephone: 800/650-6787 or 781/639-1872
Fax: 781/639-2982
E-mail: *customerservice@hcpro.com*

Visit HCPro at its World Wide Web sites:
***www.hcpro.com* and *www.hcmarketplace.com*.**

01/2005
20249

Contents

About the expert

Adrianne E. Avillion, DEd, RN

Adrianne E. Avillion, DEd, RN, is the president and owner of AEA Consulting in York, PA. She specializes in designing continuing education programs for healthcare professionals and freelance medical writing. Avillion also offers consulting services in work redesign, quality improvement, and staff development.

She has published extensively, including serving as editor of the first and second editions of *The Core Curriculum for Staff Development,* published by the National Nursing Staff Development Organization (NNSDO). She is also a frequent presenter at conferences and conventions devoted to continuing education and staff development. She was recently elected vice president of the board of directors for the NNSDO. Avillion holds a master's degree in nursing and a doctorate in adult education from Penn State University.

Nursing continuing education instruction guide

Target audience

- Registered nurses (RN)
- Licensed practical nurses (LPN)
- Licensed vocational nurses (LVN)

Statement of need

Fatigue can cause slow reaction time, forgetfulness, and degraded communication and decision-making skills—all of which hinder patient safety. This handbook will educate nurses on the signs of fatigue so they can recognize it in themselves and their coworkers and prevent further occurrences.

Educational objectives

Upon completion of this activity, participants should be able to

- define fatigue
- identify safety-related risks associated with fatigue
- identify two physical factors that impact fatigue
- list signs and symptoms of fatigue
- identify tips for combating fatigue

Faculty

Adrianne E. Avillion, DEd, RN

Accreditation/designation statement

This educational activity for one contact hour is provided by HCPro, Inc. HCPro is accredited as a provider of continuing nursing education by the American Nurses Credentialing Center's (ANCC) Commission on Accreditation.

Disclosure statement

Adrianne E. Avillion has signed a vested interest form declaring that she has no commercial/financial stake in this activity.

Instructions

In order to be eligible to receive your nursing contact hour for this activity, you are required to do the following:

1. Read the handbook
2. Complete the exam*
3. Complete the evaluation
4. Provide your contact information located on the exam and evaluation
5. Submit exam and evaluation to HCPro, Inc.

Please provide all of the information requested above and mail or fax your completed exam and evaluation to

Robin L. Flynn
Manager, Continuing Education
HCPro, Inc.
200 Hoods Lane
P.O. Box 1168
Marblehead, MA 01945
Fax: 781/639-0179

If you have any questions, please contact Robin Flynn at 781/639-1872 or *rflynn@hcpro.com.*

* If you are using this handbook for general training purposes (without offering continuing education credits), please note that the answers to the final exam questions are printed in the book *Fight Fatigue: A Nurse Manager's Guide to Reducing Risk and Revitalizing Staff,* published by HCPro, Inc.

Fight Fatigue: A Training Handbook for Nurses

Fatigue and its consequences

Why are nurses so tired? When you ask your coworkers this question, their first responses probably include phrases such as "overworked and understaffed," "too much stress," "too much overtime," or "not enough respect." These factors do indeed play a significant role in the development of fatigue, but they are not the **only** reasons that nurses are tired. The purpose of this handbook is to help you recognize fatigue, identify the obvious and hidden factors that cause it, and, most importantly, help you deal with and reduce or eliminate those situations that cause it.

What is fatigue?

Mosby's *Medical, Nursing, & Allied Health Dictionary* defines fatigue as "a state of exhaustion or a loss of strength and endurance."[1] "Fatigue" is a recognized nursing diagnosis. The Eighth National Conference on the Classification of Nursing Diagnoses defined fatigue as an "overwhelming sense of exhaustion and decreased capacity for physical and mental work regardless of adequate sleep."[2]

In other words, fatigue isn't simply feeling tired after a hard day's (or evening's or night's) work. It is an overwhelming sensation of exhaustion that can affect many, if not all, aspects of your work and home life. Fatigue, if it's severe enough and if it lasts long enough, may jeopardize careers, damage interpersonal relationships, and impair physical and psychological functioning.

Signs and symptoms

How can you help to pull yourself up and away from the adverse effects of fatigue? First, you need to be able to recognize them. Some of the signs and symptoms of fatigue are much more obvious than others. In fact, the people who complain most often and most loudly about being tired may not be suffering from the effects of fatigue as much as your colleagues who suffer in silence. How can you tell if you or one of your colleagues is fatigued? Let's discuss the most obvious signs and symptoms first.

Verbal complaints

Verbal complaints are probably the most common signs of fatigue. Comments about fatigue and exhaustion are blatant, but other, more subtle, verbal comments are just as indicative of fatigue. For example, you or your coworkers may

- talk about not having the energy to perform routine tasks at work and at home

- complain about physical ailments (e.g., headaches, backaches, nausea, diarrhea)

- discuss feelings of irritability and difficulty concentrating

- complain about not getting enough sleep or being unable to sleep

Observable signs of fatigue

What are some nonverbal signs and symptoms of fatigue that can help you recognize and deal with this problem? Let's review some observations that can indicate the existence of serious fatigue:

- Do you "look" tired? Are you pale? Are there dark circles under your eyes? Do you feel listless?

- Usually efficient in your work-related duties, are you now having difficulty completing your assignments? Do even routine tasks seem to overwhelm you? Are you the last to leave after your shifts are completed because you need to "catch up" on charting and other non-direct patient care tasks?

- Have you used more sick time recently? Do you seem to be unusually susceptible to colds, flu, and other illnesses?

- Are you suddenly accident-prone? Are you having difficulty concentrating?

- Has there been an increase in the occurrence of medical errors?
- Are you unusually emotionally labile?
- Are you not interested in activities and projects about which you are normally enthused?
- Are you concerned about your interpersonal relationships? Are you experiencing a decrease in libido?

The impact of fatigue: Evidence-based data

Research shows that when and for how long you work contribute to fatigue and, consequently, to the occurrence of medical errors. Stress, whether work-related or home-related, also contributes to fatigue and to the possibility of errors. The following information is based on research conducted on fatigue, its causes, and its link to medical errors.

University of Pennsylvania

University of Pennsylvania nursing professors conducted one of the first national studies to examine the effects of long work hours and fatigue on the job performance of nurses. Published in the July/August 2004 issue of *Health Affairs,* this study reviewed the work habits of 393 hospital staff nurses. These nurses, through the use of logbooks, tracked hours worked, overtime, days off, and their sleeping patterns for 28 days. Participants also described errors or "near" errors during their time at work.[3]

According to the participants' logbook recordings, 199 errors were committed and 213 near-errors occurred during the 28-day investigative period. The majority of the errors (58%) dealt with medication administration. Other errors included the following:

- Errors of procedure (18%)
- Errors of documentation (12%)
- Errors of transcription (7%)

The findings from this study suggest that the routine use of 12-hour shifts should be reduced and that the use of overtime as a compensation for staffing shortages increases the possibility of error.[4]

Agency for Healthcare Research and Quality

Healthcare professionals must use sound judgment when making clinical assessments and react swiftly and accurately during emergencies, often making life or death decisions under conditions of extreme stress. Fatigue can impair judgment and decision-making skills, thus compromising patient safety.

An Agency for Healthcare Research and Quality (AHRQ) report, published in 2004, investigated how sleepiness and fatigue affect patient safety.[5] The majority of experts agree that adults require between six and 10 hours of sleep per 24 hours, and most adults need about eight hours of sleep per day. Research also shows that when adults get less than five hours of sleep per 24 hours, mental abilities start to show impairment. If you are getting at least four hours of sleep for a limited amount of time (e.g., two to three days), you are probably still able to function at a reasonable level of safety but below your normal level of activity. However, if sleep deprivation is an ongoing problem, individuals develop what is called sleep debt. Sleep debt leads to a significant reduction in general performance, alertness, and response time as well as causing changes in mood, motivation, initiative, and morale according to the AHRQ report.

Effects of shift rotation

Shift rotation and the frequency or pattern of shift rotation also contribute to fatigue. Shift workers experience circadian rhythm disturbances, have poorer sleep quality compared to those persons who do not rotate shifts, experience less rapid eye movement (REM) sleep, and are more likely to complain of sleepiness after awakening and during work hours. Additionally, research shows that sleep after working night shifts is generally shorter than sleep after working day shifts. All of these factors contribute to sleep deprivation, as indicated by less alertness during night work and a reduction in reasoning ability, the report said.

The method or timing of shift rotation and the speed with which rotation occurs can also impact performance. For example, nurses who rotate morning shifts, then evening shifts, then night shifts (referred to as "forward" rotation) generally experience less fatigue than those who rotate "backward" from day shift to night shift to evening shift. This trend is believed to be due to circadian rhythms, which tend to move forward. Several studies support forward rotation, but two studies found no significant changes in fatigue levels in a comparison of forward and backward rotation, said the AHRQ. Further investigation is needed to determine validity and reliability pertaining to this issue.

The report also suggests that gradually changing from one shift to another (e.g., rotating shifts every one to two weeks) may allow for easier adaptation of circadian rhythm than does following a more rapid rotation (e.g., rotating shifts every two to three days). A slow shift rotation allows for longer length of sleep at home, less sleepiness at work, and fewer errors.

Physical factors that cause fatigue

Nurses seem particularly vulnerable to back, leg, and foot problems due to the physical requirements of bedside nursing. Problems in these areas increase the incidence and intensity of fatigue. What can you do to alleviate such difficulties?

1. Wear good support hose to enhance circulation and reduce fatigue. Knee socks under pant uniforms seem to be particularly popular, but they can impede circulation as they press into the calf muscles. Instead, properly fitting support hose can help to reduce debilitating fatigue.

2. Wear shoes that provide proper support. If you don't, that could be another source of fatigue. In addition, nurses should not wear the same pair of shoes two days in row because shoes need time to "breathe" and dry out before being worn again.

3. Consider the health of your feet. Corns, bunions, and other foot problems can make walking difficult and painful and can actually make you tire more quickly. Therefore, seek medical attention for any such problems as soon as possible.

Achilles tendonitis

Do you maintain a regular exercise regimen or are you actively involved in sports? You may be in danger of developing Achilles tendonitis, a painful and often debilitating inflammation of the Achilles tendon. This condition may result from a single incident of aggravating the tendon or from a series of actions that place stress on the tendon, causing small tears to develop over time. The following are risk factors in the development of Achilles tendonitis:

- Activities that require sudden starts and stops and repetitive jumping. Examples include basketball, tennis, dancing, and running.

- Wearing inappropriate footwear when participating in the aforementioned activities.

- Lack of flexibility in muscles and tendons. This is often a problem for persons who exercise infrequently or who are just starting an exercise or sports regimen.

- High-heeled shoes. When high heels are worn, the Achilles tendon (and leg muscles) adapt to a shortened position because such shoes prevent the heel from stretching appropriately to the ground. When people switch to sneakers (or other footwear worn by nurses at work), the tendon must stretch further than it is accustomed to stretching and inflammation occurs.

Flat feet

Flat feet is a common problem characterized by a flattening out of the arch of the foot and is also referred to as a fallen arch. Although this condition generally does not cause significant problems, it can sometimes contribute to or aggravate other foot problems. And how can you tell that significant foot problems are present? Consider consulting a podiatrist if you have one or more of the following conditions:

- Your feet hurt. Feet should not hurt, and pain is the body's way of letting you know that something is wrong.
- You experience pain in your shins.
- You have "weak" ankles or often sprain your ankles.
- You experience chronic lower-back, heel, or knee pain.
- Your toes do not appear to be straight.
- One side of the soles of your shoes wears out more quickly than the other side.
- When you walk your feet point inward or excessively outward.

A possible solution for some of these problems is to use orthotics, which help to treat or adjust various mechanical foot problems. Some orthotics, which include such items as cushioned heel cups or insoles to place in your shoes, can be purchased over-the-counter in drug stores. Others are custom-made, designed to meet the specific needs of a particular individual. The latter are considerably more expensive.

Back pain

Using proper equipment (such as lifting and positioning devices), sitting in ergonomically correct chairs, wearing back support braces, and using proper body mechanics when lifting and positioning are obvious measures to take in order to avoid back injuries. However, many (if not most) nurses lift and position patients without help because "we're short staffed" or "everyone else is busy." You must learn to take care of yourself and help take care of your colleagues by helping them perform difficult tasks, such as lifting and positioning.

CASE STUDY #1

Q **You are a busy nurse on a pediatric unit. You are also slightly overweight. You recently enrolled in a weight-loss program, sponsored by your hospital, that includes taking nutritional supplements and regular exercise. You've lost some weight and have more energy than you did prior to starting the program. However, after about four weeks, you begin to have trouble sleeping. The insomnia is starting to worry you and you begin to feel tired at work. What might be causing your sleep disturbance?**

A Assuming that there are no underlying physical or mental illnesses, look at the components of the weight-loss program. Exercise programs are great, but did you consult your healthcare provider first? No one should initiate a program without such a discussion. When are you exercising? Is it right before bedtime? If so, it will interfere with your ability to sleep. Finally, what's in that nutritional supplement? Many weight-loss products contain large amounts of caffeine. Check the ingredients.

Sleep disorders

Adequate sleep and rest are necessary if the body is to remain healthy and function normally. Lack of sleep contributes to the fatigue that interferes with normal activities of daily living, including job performance. Most adults need between eight and 10 hours of sleep per day. According to the National Institute of Neurological Disorders and Stroke, about 40 million Americans experience some type of chronic long-term sleep disorder annually. An additional 20 million Americans experience sporadic sleep disorders.[6] Sleep disorders fall into three broad categories:

- **Insomnia**—Defined as the inability to fall asleep. Persons who experience insomnia feel tired most of the time and often worry about not getting enough sleep.

- **Disturbed sleep**—Characterized by interrupted sleep patterns. Sleep apnea is a type of disturbed sleep that occurs when the person experiences a temporary cessation of breathing, or apnea, during sleep.

- **Increased sleep**—Narcolepsy, for example, causes people to fall asleep abruptly and without warning or control.

Causes of sleep disorders

Both physical and mental illnesses can contribute to sleep disorders. In fact, almost all persons suffering from mental health problems also experience sleep disorders. Stress also has a profound effect on sleep patterns. An issue that is of particular interest to nurses and others who work alternate shifts is Night Shift Sleep Disorder.

Some of the research findings on shift work and fatigue show that the direction and swiftness of shift rotation contribute to fatigue. Night Shift Sleep Disorder is the result of changes in the biological "clock" and circadian rhythms caused by shift work. These rhythms control the way we function physically and mentally during a single 24-hour period. For most of us, darkness often triggers drowsiness and prepares us for sleep. For persons working nights and evenings, however, the rest of the world is asleep while they must function at their best. Some research indicates that night shift workers have higher incidences of heart disease, digestive difficulties, and experience more emotional and mental health problems than those who work during the day.

Treatment of sleep disorders

What can you do to cope with sleep disorders? For those employees who work nights and evenings, try to work a forward rotation (e.g., days to evenings, to nights) and avoid rotating shifts too often. Some research findings suggest that working a particular shift for about two weeks allows the body time to adapt. What else can you do to promote better sleep? Here are some ideas:

- **Have a thorough physical and mental health exam.** If an underlying cause such as a physical or mental illness is causing or contributing to sleep problems, the illness must be diagnosed and treated.

- **Examine medication regimens.** Have you added to or deleted from your regimen any medications? Don't forget that this includes not only prescription drugs but also over-the-counter medications, herbal preparations, vitamins and minerals, nutritional supplements, and weight-loss products.

- **Don't exercise right before bed.** Exercise regularly, but not near bedtime.

- **Examine your leisure habits.** How much caffeine do you ingest? How much alcohol do you drink? Do you abuse drugs such as prescription (e.g., pain medication, sleeping pills) or illegal substances?

- **Establish a schedule for sleep.** Try to go to bed and get up at the same time every day.

- **Prepare your sleeping environment.** Make sure that your bedroom is dark, especially if you must sleep during the day. Hang curtains that effectively block light or purchase a sleep mask that covers your eyes.

- **Establish a relaxing bedtime ritual.** Include taking a hot bath or shower, reading a book, or listening to soothing music. Note that a bath is more conducive to sleep than a shower, which generally stimulates rather than relaxes.

- **Clear your mind.** Do not attempt to sleep while thinking about problems at work or at home. This can be quite a challenge, but try to clear your mind. There are a variety of inexpensive audiotapes and CDs that offer music composed specifically to induce sleep and relaxation.

- **Resolve conflict.** Try not to go to bed angry with work colleagues or with family. Do your best to resolve such issues prior to attempting to sleep.

Psychosocial causes of fatigue

Psychosocial issues that can lead to serious fatigue include stress, depression, and generalized anxiety disorder (GAD). Although these issues are not the only factors that contribute to fatigue, they are the ones occurring with increasing frequency in the United States. By reviewing and understanding the issues described in this section, you will be better prepared to recognize and investigate additional psychosocial matters that affect you and, consequently, your job performance.

Stress

Stress is a response to a specific event or state of events—positive or negative—that affects a person's physical, psychological, or emotional well-being.

Personal stress: Many people believe that personal stress is only caused by negative events in our lives, such as death of a loved one, financial problems, substance abuse, or marital discord, but research shows that even joyous events such as the birth of a much-wanted child, a wedding, or a busy holiday season can produce damaging amounts of stress.

Occupational stress: Occupational or job-related stress is defined as the "harmful emotional and physical reactions resulting from the interactions between the worker and her or his work environment where the demands of the job exceed the worker's capabilities and resources."[7] Some sources of job-related stress are common among many professions. Others are unique to nursing. But even universal stressors such as conflicts with coworkers and increased workload are generally more intense in the healthcare setting because employees in these settings are responsible for the lives of fellow human beings.

Because nurses as a group focus particularly on providing support and care to others and are quick to ignore their own needs, they may feel guilty about reacting negatively to an event that they believe should be totally positive (e.g., holiday plans, child bearing, etc.).[8] Therefore, even though nurses often do a good job recognizing the signs of stress, especially if they believe that they are wrong to feel that way, they need help and support in dealing with all types of stressors. Part of providing such help is to avoid criticizing someone for what you may perceive as an overreaction. Such criticism will only increase the stress and ultimately have a negative impact on organizational performance.

Depression

Depression is characterized by feelings of sadness that can not be explained by the sufferer. Depressed persons experience a significant decrease in energy, an increase in fatigue, and a lack of interest in activities that normally bring them pleasure. Depression can also lead to impaired functioning at work, at home, and in social situations. Here are some statistics that may help you to assess the possibility of depression in yourself or your coworkers:

- Depression occurs at any age, but onset most often takes place in persons 24–44 years of age.

- Major depressive disorder is more common among women. It affects 20% of women and 10% of men.

- Depression is diagnosed more often in Caucasians from middle- and upper-class families. This may be due to the fact that persons from lower socioeconomic backgrounds are less able to afford the cost of seeking medical help for symptoms of depression.

- The most common cause of a depressive episode in adults is the death of a spouse.

- Women are at higher risk for depression during pregnancy and within the first few months after giving birth.

Generalized anxiety disorder (GAD)

All of us experience anxiety at one time or another. Anxiety is a normal response to dangerous, stressful, or uncertain situations. However, persons suffering from GAD experience pathological anxiety that is excessive and chronic. Such anxiety is out of proportion with the stressors in their lives and interferes with their ability to perform their normal activities of daily living. GAD can be a debilitating problem and can impair the ability to function at work, at home, and in social situations.

GAD is not an easy disorder to understand. Family, friends, and coworkers may become inpatient with and contemptuous of someone who "worries all of the time." However, people who suffer from GAD need medical help and support from family, friends, and coworkers in order to overcome its negative impact.

CASE STUDY #2

Q **After seeking help for her depression from your hospital's employee health program, your colleague Sandra is now taking the antidepressant Zoloft. After six months of medication therapy, her depression has lifted significantly. In the past month, however, she tells you that she's been drowsy at work and has suffered from headaches and tremors. She tells you that she knows these can be side effects of Zoloft, so she is thinking of discontinuing it. She also tells you that she began taking an herbal supplement, St. John's wort, about a month ago because "it's supposed to help with depression." How does this combination impact fatigue?**

A Herbs can interact adversely with other herbs or medications. In this case, St. John's wort should not be taken in conjunction with Zoloft because it can increase the effects of the prescribed medication and increase the possibility of serotonin syndrome. This case illustrates how even well-educated healthcare professionals can make errors in self-medication. Recognize that such errors can jeopardize your (or your coworkers') heath and well-being—as well as your job performance.

Complementary approaches to fighting fatigue

In this section, we will provide an overview of complementary approaches to addressing fatigue and its various causes. It is not intended as a substitute for adequate medical evaluation and intervention. Here are a few precautions to keep in mind when evaluating complementary medicine:

- Talk to your physician about any complementary approaches you are using or thinking about using. Some of these approaches, such as herbal medicines, can interact dangerously with other herbs, vitamins, nutritional supplements, and prescription and over-the-counter medications.

- Being labeled "natural" does not necessarily mean that a given approach is safe.

- Purchase herbs and other supplements only from reliable manufacturing companies.

- Report to your healthcare provider any side effects of complementary approaches

Many techniques require instruction or intervention by qualified teachers or therapists. However, one advantage to some complementary medicine approaches is that they can be implemented rapidly with little risk. For example, if you and your colleagues are experiencing work-related stress because of short-staffing, you can learn and implement such "stress-busters" as guided imagery, meditation, and relaxation breathing techniques. Also consider the following interventions:

- **Exercise:** When you are tired and stressed, exercise may be the last thing you may want to do, but the ultimate benefits of exercise are well worth the effort. Participating in an aerobic exercise program for 20–30 minutes a day, five days a week can increase energy and reduce stress.

- **Tai chi chuan, or tai chi:** This an ancient form of martial art and meditation that combines a series of slow physical movements with meditation, mental concentration, and coordinated breathing. Research indicates that tai chi improves endurance, flexibility, muscle tone, and balance. It can help you to improve awareness of your mind and body and stop worries, sadness, and anxiety from dominating.

- **Yoga:** A number of studies have shown that yoga helps to alleviate stress and anxiety, lowers blood pressure, relieves pain, improves metabolic and respiratory function, improves motor skills, and enhances relaxation.

Herbal therapy

About 80% of the world's population use herbs or other nutritional supplements for medicinal purposes. However, almost 75% of these people never tell their healthcare providers that they do so.[9] This can cause serious problems and even fatal reactions or interactions with other herbs, nutritional supplements, prescription drugs, or over-the-counter medications. For example, a patient may read or hear that garlic can lower cholesterol, so he or she begins to ingest large amounts of garlic tablets. This may not cause a problem, but garlic has anticoagulant properties, so if such a patient is taking an anticoagulant prescription medication as well, dangerous bleeding problems may occur. Herbs used to alleviate

- fatigue include bee pollen, cola, ginseng, and yerba mate
- anxiety include chamomile, kava, and lemon balm
- depression include ginkgo, hops, mistletoe, and St. John's wort

References

1. Anderson, D.M. (Chief Lexicographer), *Mosby's Medical, Nursing, and Allied Health Directory, 6th ed.,* (St. Louis: 2002).

2. American Federation of Teachers. (2001). *Long work hours for nurses linked to medical errors.* Retrieved December 1, 2004, from *www.aft.org/healthcare/news/errors.htm.*

3. Medical News Service. (2004). *Grand valley state university study finds connection between nurse fatigue, patient errors.* Retrieved November 23, 2004, from *www.medicalnewsservice.com/fullstory.cfm?storyID=2330&fback+yes.*

4. See note 3 above.

5. Jha, A. K., Duncan, B. W., and Bates, D. W. (2004). *Chapter 46. Fatigue, sleepiness, and medical errors.* Taken from *Evidence Report/Technology Assessment, No. 43 Making Health Care Safer: A Critical Analysis of*

6. Neurology Channel. (2004). *Sleep disorders.* Retrieved December 13, 2004, from *www.neurologychannel.com/sleepdisorders.*

7. International Council of Nurses. (2004). *ICN on occupational stress and the threat to worker health.* Retrieved December 1, 2004, from *www.icn.ch/matters_stress_print.htm.*

8. Phillips, K. (2003). "Nurses too focused on the giving in caregiving for their own good." Retrieved December 21, 2004, from *www.nursezone.com/include/PrintArticle.asp?articleid=11442&Profile=For%20You.*

9. Kelly, W. J. (Editorial Director). (2004). *Nursing 2004 herbal medicine handbook (2nd ed.).* Philadelphia: Lippincott Williams & Wilkins.

Nursing education exam
Fight Fatigue: A Training Handbook for Nurses

Name: ______________________________

Title: ______________________________

Facility name: ______________________________

Address: ______________________________

Address: ______________________________

City: ____________________ **State:** ______ **ZIP:** __________

Phone number: ______________________________

Fax number: ______________________________

E-mail: ______________________________

Nursing license number: ______________________________

(ANCC requires a unique identifier for each learner)

1. **Fatigue can impair nurses' judgment and decision-making skills, causing all of the following EXCEPT**

    a. compromised patient safety
    b. more efficient patient care
    c. extra charting time
    d. conflicts with management

2. **Which of the following may be a subtle sign that one of your coworkers is suffering from fatigue?**

    a. Gossip about patients and management
    b. Talking excessively about sexual activities
    c. Hyperactivity
    d. Discussions about not having the energy to perform routine tasks at work and at home

3. All of the following could be symptoms of fatigue EXCEPT

a. routine assignments are still easy to complete
b. you are unusually susceptible colds, flu, and other illnesses
c. you find yourself suddenly accident-prone
d. lack of interest in activities about which you are normally enthused

4. A University of Pennsylvania study published in 2004, which examined the effects of long work hours and fatigue on job performance, revealed that during the 28-day investigative period, the largest percentage of the nurses 199 errors and 213 near-errors had to do with _____.

a. equipment use
b. documentation
c. patient education
d. medication administration

5. Research shows that when adults get less than ____ hours of sleep per 24 hours, mental abilities start to show impairment.

a. 8
b. 7
c. 5
d. 10

6. The method or timing of shift rotation and the speed with which rotation occurs can also impact performance. What do researchers suggest for lessening the effects of shift rotation on fatigue?

a. Always rotate "backward" from night shift to night shift to morning shift
b. Gradually change from one shift to another (e.g., rotating shifts every one to two weeks)
c. Rotate shifts rapidly (e.g., every two to three days)
d. Sleep in a room that receives plenty of natural light

7. **Achilles tendonitis is a painful and often debilitating inflammation of the Achilles tendon to which you may be vulnerable if you participate in activities that require sudden starts and stops (e.g., dancing, tennis), have a lack of flexibility in your muscles and tendons, or ______________________.**

    a. wear high-heeled shoes frequently and switch to sneakers for your shift
    b. suffer from a chronic illness such as diabetes
    c. don't soak your feet before and after your shift
    d. walk to work everyday

8. **________________ is the result of changes in the biological "clock" and circadian rhythms caused by shift work.**

    a. Insomnia
    b. Night Shift Sleep Disorder
    c. Disturbed sleep
    d. Sleep debt

9. **Getting a thorough physical and mental health exam, establishing a relaxing bedtime ritual, and ________________ are all things you can do to promote better sleep.**

    a. examining your medication regimen for new prescriptions, vitamins, weight-loss products, etc.
    b. exercising right before you go to bed
    c. staggering the times you wake up
    d. staggering the times you go to sleep

10. **A nurse with whom family, friends, and coworkers have become impatient and contemptuous because he or she "worries all of the time" may be suffering from _____.**

    a. self-pity
    b. worry-wart syndrome
    c. a lack of initiative
    d. generalized anxiety disorder (GAD)

Nursing education evaluation
Fight Fatigue: A Training Handbook for Nurses

Name: ______________________________

Title: ______________________________

Facility name: ______________________________

Address: ______________________________

Address: ______________________________

City: ____________________ **State:** ______ **ZIP:** __________

Phone number: ______________________________

Fax number: ______________________________

E-mail: ______________________________

Nursing license number: ______________________________

(ANCC requires a unique identifier for each learner)

	Strongly Agree	Agree	Disagree	Strongly Disagree
1. Please indicate below how well you feel this activity met the learning objectives listed. Please provide a response for each learning objective. At the end of this activity I will be able to				
define fatigue	1	2	3	4
identify safety-related risks associated with fatigue	1	2	3	4
identify two physical factors that impact fatigue	1	2	3	4
list signs and symptoms of fatigue	1	2	3	4
identify tips for combating fatigue	1	2	3	4
2. Objectives were related to the overall purpose/goal of the activity	1	2	3	4

	Strongly Agree	Agree	Disagree	Strongly Disagree
3. The exam for the activity was an accurate test of the knowledge gained	1	2	3	4
4. The activity avoided commercial bias or influence	1	2	3	4

5. Will this learning activity enhance your professional nursing practice?

❑ Yes ❑ No

6. How committed are you to making the behavioral changes suggested in this activity?

❑ Very Committed ❑ Somewhat Committed ❑ Not Committed

7. Please provide us with your degree

❑ ADN ❑ BSN ❑ MSN ❑ Other ________________

8. Please provide us with your credentials

❑ LVN ❑ LPN ❑ RN ❑ NP ❑ Other ________________

9. I found the process to obtain my continuing education credits for this activity easy to complete

Strongly Agree Agree Disagree Strongly Disagree

10. If you did not find the process easy to complete, please state why.

____

11. Providing nursing contact hours on this activity influenced my decision to participate.

Strongly Agree Agree Disagree Strongly Disagree

12. How much time did it take for you to complete this activity?

____

13. Would you be interested in participating as a pilot tester for the development of future HCPro nursing education activities?

❑ Yes ❑ No

Thank you for completing this evaluation of our nursing CE activity!